Beauty for the Busy Woman

The Six Day Program for the Busy Woman

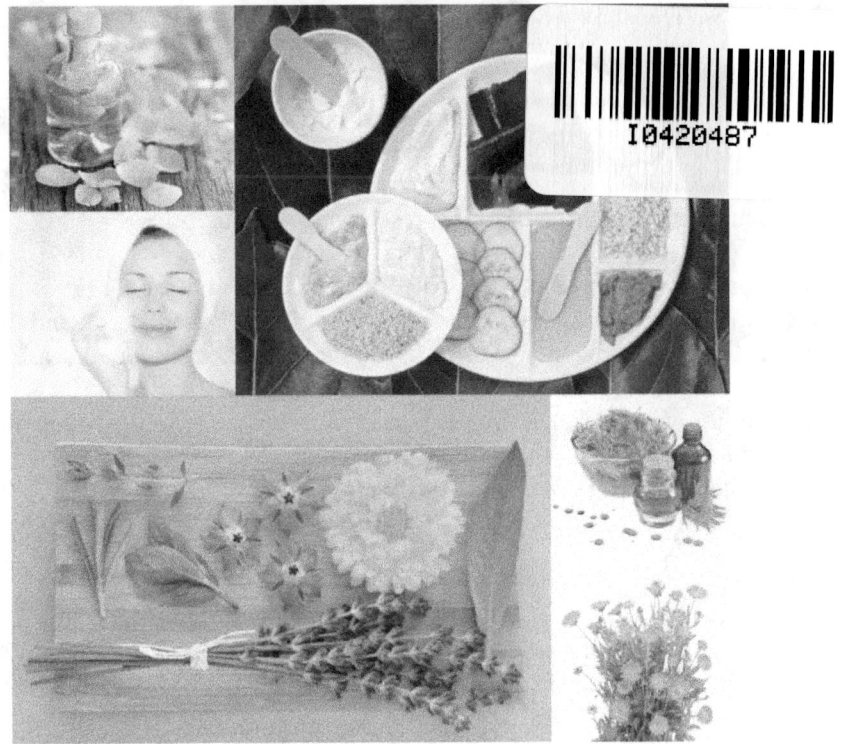

Health Learning Series
Dueep Jyot Singh
Mendon Cottage Books

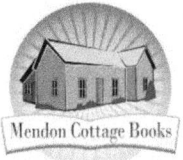

JD-Biz Publishing
Download Free Books!

http://MendonCottageBooks.com

Disclaimer

The information is this book is provided for informational purposes only. It is not intended to be used and medical advice or a substitute for proper medical treatment by a qualified health care provider. The information is believed to be accurate as presented based on research by the author.

The contents have not been evaluated by the U.S. Food and Drug Administration or any other Government or Health Organization and the contents in this book are not to be used to treat cure or prevent disease.

The author or publisher is not responsible for the use or safety of any diet, procedure or treatment mentioned in this book. The author or publisher is not responsible for errors or omissions that may exist.

Warning

The Book is for informational purposes only and before taking on any diet, treatment or medical procedure it is recommended to consult with your primary health care provider.

Download Free Books!

http://MendonCottageBooks.com

Table of Contents

Introduction

There was a time when I was so busy that my getting ready schedule on a hectic morning took anywhere between 7 to 10 minutes. And when I asked one of my equally busy colleagues, if she could take some time out, to a spa for the weekend for a little bit of pampering, because we needed it, this was her answer.

"Oh, do me a favor, DJ. Who really has the time to spend trying to beautify herself at home, or in a spa, when one does not even have the time to lie down and expire peacefully. Cannot you see that we are so busy the whole day long that if you imagine we have a few minutes for ourselves that in itself is a blessing. I am not going to be spending that time pampering myself and beautifying myself when I would rather be lying face down on a couch, fast asleep."

Women have got so into the habit of being busy, busy, busy that they have forgotten the idea of cherishing themselves. How many times have you heard this statement, that one is so busy that one really does not have the time for "beautifying" one. In fact, many women I know use this as a very convenient excuse to look dowdy, and badly groomed. Because they are under the impression that good grooming takes a lot of time, and this should be done only on very special occasions. I beg to differ.

A woman who does not take some time off to cherish and cosset herself is either lacking in self-esteem, or does not seem to have any interest in the mere fact that she is fortunate to have been born a woman.

But then, many of us are going to say who really has the time and energy to spend long periods of time beautifying one when it is go go go from early morning till night. Yes, everybody knows that at the end of the day, a woman would like nothing better than to kick off her shoes, snuggle down in a comfortable sofa close her eyes and think deep deep, deep thoughts.

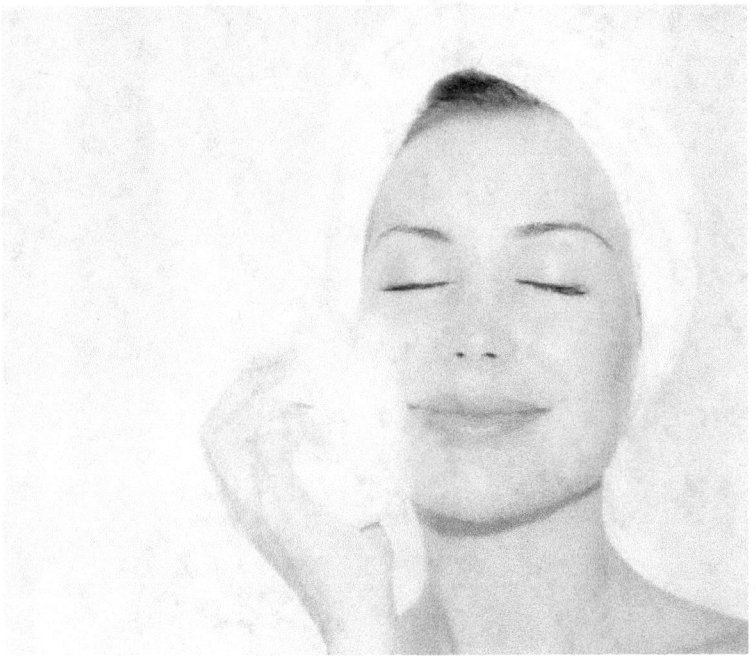

So let us start a six-day beauty program with just thinking, and eyes closed.

Firstly, let us start with relaxation. Unfortunately, the number of workaholics is increasing, because women have decided that more money in hand is their top priority. They are more focused on their family's future financial security and so naturally they are not going to spend their time and hard-earned money in long winded beauty treatments in Salons and spas. Also, these women with hectic and busy schedules have forgotten how to relax.

So before we start on our six-day beauty treatment, here are some points, which you have to implement every day, to stay beautiful and stay healthy. Many of them are commonsense tips, but how many of us implement them in real life? *We do not have the time…*

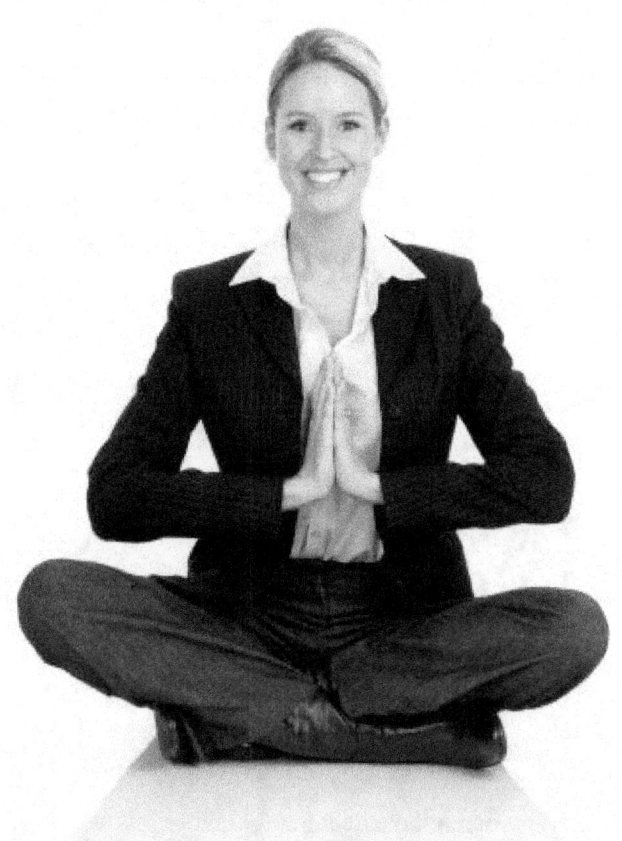

It is hard for a busy woman to take some time out of a busy schedule to pamper herself.

Take a deep breath and let your muscles hang loose. Now stretch yourself slowly, just like a cat does. In fact, I do the stretching exercise the moment I wake up, to straighten out the kinks in my neck and back, as well as getting my muscles into action mode. I find that the stretching exercise done first thing in the morning is quite enough to keep me in a good and happy state of mind throughout the day.

How many glasses of water have you drunk through the day? Compare them with how many cups of coffee have you drunk instead? If you are a coffee addict, sorry I cannot help you, but try substituting coffee for fresh fruit juice and water. Caffeine addicts are going to find themselves unable to wean themselves from this addiction, but caffeine is one thing which gives you sleepless nights. And sleepless nights are not conducive to good health and beauty. Besides, believe me, fresh fruit juice is going to give you such a wonderful glow to your skin that you are going to wonder why you never tried it before.

A normally liquid intake must be between one and 1.5 L, so as to keep your body from dehydrating. If you have time enough before running to that early morning meeting or anything else planned for the day, drink a glass of cucumber, orange or tomato juice. These have to be freshly made, no concentrates, please. That is a fine way to give you an instant healthy energy boost.

To begin your beauty regime with that glow to your complexion, try this new formula and come back to nature. We do have very good soaps, creams and other chemical-based beauty formulations which are good enough to make you feel that you are looking your best. But all these chemicals and lanolin-based creams spoils the natural composition of your skin and its texture.

You may touch your skin and find it soft and smooth and silky. But in the long run, the natural oils secreted from the skin get covered up with lanolin. This may lead to the clogging of pores, resulting in small pimples and blackheads. Strangely enough, people never think of blaming expensive creams and lotions for skin problems.

Many beauty consultants recommend a constant cleansing of the face to keep a smooth skin. And then they recommend a natural skin cleanser and moisturizer. What they are not going to tell you is that there is only going to be one natural ingredient extract in that expensive skin cleanser and moisturizer. And you buy it, and you are impressed with its short-term results. But soon you find yourself with a wrinkled skin. That is the long-term side effect of the chemicals on your skin.

Women in old times, kept their peaches and cream complexion by using homemade soap and hot water to cleanse off the grime and dirt of the day. But at that time, the atmosphere was not contaminated with harmful pollutants and the water did not have poisonous chemicals pumped into it. Unfortunately, that is one of the side effects of progress in the 21st century. So if you can manage to clean your face with warm water, which has cooled off after boiling, so much the better. At least some of the pollutants have been eliminated. The best water, of course, is rainwater collected *after the first showers.* The first showers are going to be heavily polluted with the chemical pollutants in the atmosphere and air. So if it is raining heavily and has been doing so for the last 4 to 5 minutes, go outside with a couple of utensils and place them in an area where there is no dust or dirt. This rainwater is soft, and excellent for your complexion. Just bottle it and use whenever you need it.

Use chemical-based soaps to the bare minimum. I am going to give you recipes for natural cleansers further on. Also, the best way to clean up those clogged up pores is to keep a bottle of cucumber juice in your bag and readily accessible. During your lunch break, you can always clean your face with a bit of cotton dipped in this cucumber juice. It freshens up your face wonderfully. Cucumber juice has been used since ancient times to reduce wrinkles and for cleaning up all the dust and grime accumulated during the day.

Day One – This is going to be detoxifying and natural bleaching day

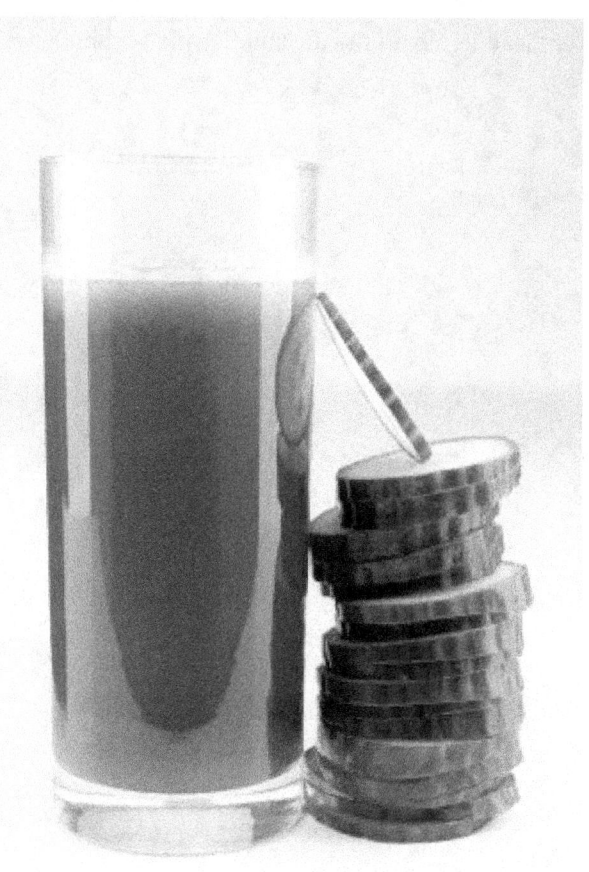

Drink fresh cucumber juice, as well as apply it all over your body, as many times as you can during the day.

If you have some free time during the day, apply a cucumber facemask. This is going to be made up of grated cucumber, Fuller salt, honey and a little bit of milk cream. Mix these ingredients together to make a paste. Apply this mixture all over your face, put your feet up and listen to your favorite music for the next 20 minutes. Not only is this going to clear and clean your skin, but it is going to tone it and moisturize it. Cucumbers slices all over your eyes are going to relax them.

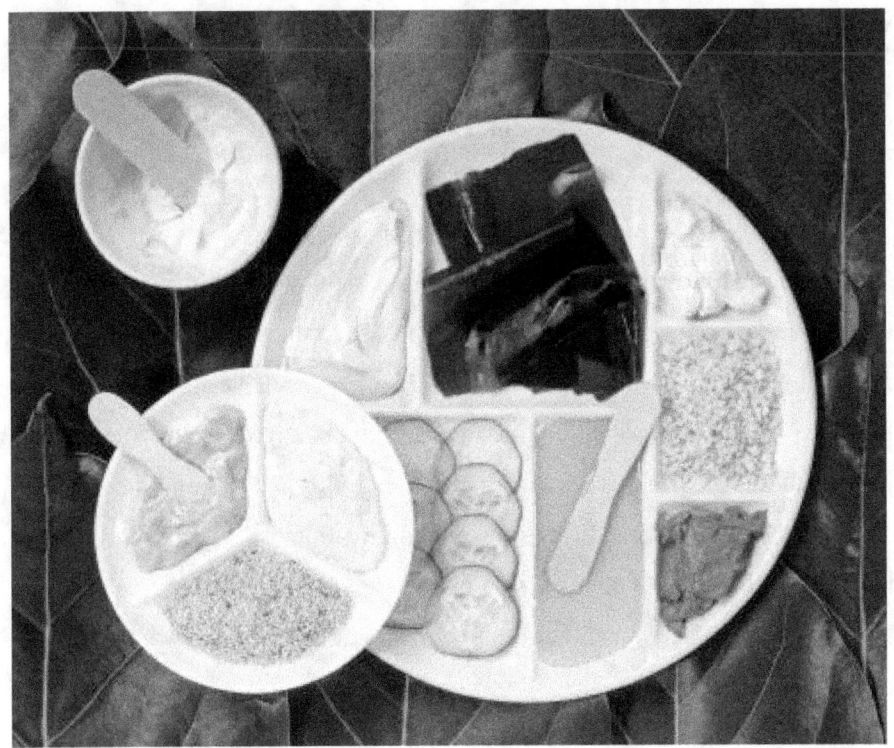

Many of the common ingredients for face mask include honey, vegetable oil, oatmeal or fullers salt and the main fruit or vegetable.

At night, if you are still looking for the peaches and cream tint to your skin, which you so often see an envy, bleach your face with a little milk cream with half a teaspoonful of cooking salt added to it. Lovely Swedish and

Scandinavian women [think Ingrid Bergman, Greta Garbo, Anita Ekberg, Ann-Margret, Britt Ekland… Busy busy busy women all, but beautiful!] swear by this treatment to keep their skin, glowing and milky white. They apply this bleacher every night without fail. Not only does this remove the dust and grime of the day, but the salt is a natural bleaching ingredient. You can either leave this mixture on, after it has been absorbed, if you are not very worried about grease stains on the bed sheets. I normally rub it off after 30 minutes, to get rid of the dead epidermal cells, and then dab cucumber juice which is easily absorbed to close the pores and to revive my skin.

See mama, no creams!

I know a little bit of sunburn looks good, especially when it gives that extra Golden tint to your skin, but too much exposure to the sun is going to destroy all of the delicacy of your skin's texture. People say it is very fashionable to be all suntanned. These people find themselves looking for beauty remedies to prevent all those wrinkles when they reach their 40s and 50s and they are the ones using chemical-based skin rejuvenating treatments like Botox. If they had treated their skin with a little bit of more loving care in their 20s and 30s and had not let it got so sunburnt, they would not be suffering from skin problems later on in life.

Let the all yummy brown and tanned sunburnt prerogative be left to men, who positively enjoy going out in the sun. They could not care less about sunburn, because their skin can take it. But you being a woman have a naturally and genetically inherited comparatively dainty skin composition. You should also remember that too much exposure to the sun can leave your skin dehydrated. And that is going to cause too many wrinkles when your dried skin starts to "pucker and wrinkle up". Nevertheless, if you have managed to catch that bit of sun during the day, a piece of potato, freshly cut and rubbed all over the sunburnt skin is going to bleach you out immediately. So day one means getting to know more about skin care, and detoxification, which is going to give you a healthy and glowing skin and Constitution.

Day 2

Today, day two in our six-day beauty regime is going to be tomato –on-skin day and hand and neck care day.

Take tomato juice in the morning and rub the pulp all over your face and body. This is an excellent exfoliating material that just gathers away dead skin and sloughs it away. Leave it on for about 20 minutes till the pulp dries. Then rub the dried pulp off and wash with warm water.

But do be careful and do not overdo the rubbing, especially if your skin is sensitive. I once found myself with zero pores, but with the red "Raw looking" skin by rubbing a bit too vigorously. From then on, I just rub gently so that the pulp is removed and then dip a cotton ball in ice water to close the pores immediately.

Now is the time to look at your hands and neck. The easiest way to keep a natural wrinkle free Look around your neck and lower portion of your chin is to massage it gently by lifting your face and looking at the roof and massaging your neck with strokes going from throat to chin.

I am going to make sure that I never have a double chin when I am in my 50s and 60s by doing this stroking massage procedure when I am bleaching my face with creamy milk and salt every night. Not only is this a good way to moisturize my neck, but it makes sure that if I neglected to rub any parts of my neck during the daily hot shower and some vestiges of dirt remained, they would be removed during this stroking and massage and cleansing process.

I have found another perfect moisturizing agent – coconut oil. Wheat germ oil and almond oil is also perfect, but as it is rather expensive and difficult to find in some of the more remote areas of Asia, plenty of Asians use coconut oil.

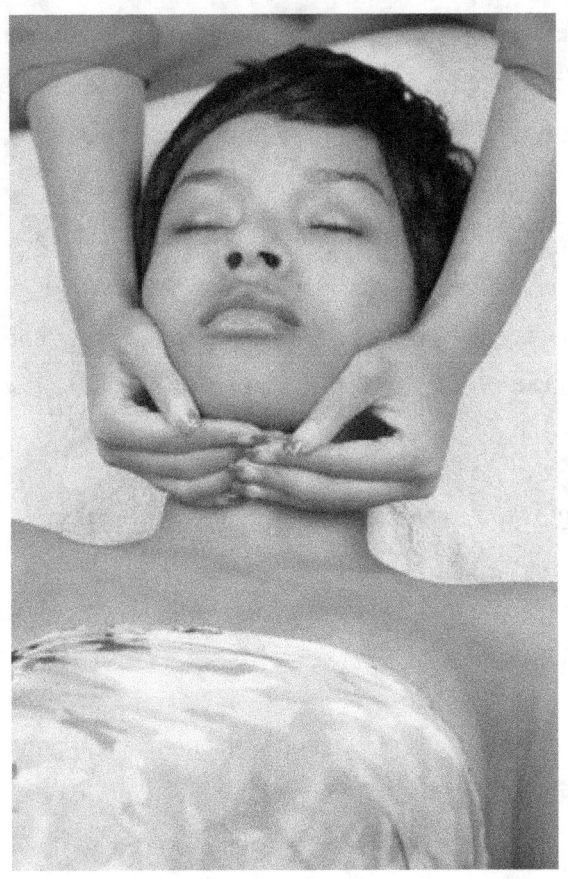

Never stroke towards the heart.

Remember that coconut oil is an acquired taste or smell. It is rather strong, but it is one of the most powerful of natural moisturizers out there. So if you find a place where you can get unrefined coconut oil, well, you are lucky, because you have a natural moisturize or for your skin, and a perfect conditioner for your hair. Well-oiled hair with the use of coconut oil will leave it tangle free throughout the week till your next shampoo.

If you have ever travelled to the mysterious Orient and have admired the rich glowing blemish free dusky complexions of many of the lovelies, and ask them the secret of their flawless glow, a large percentage will say "coconut oil." Now here is something surprising. An Oriental beauty will admit "coconut oil" to another Oriental beauty, but let any Occidental beauty ask this secret of them and they'll get an answer of "Almond oil" or "Olive oil." I wonder why that is so? It seems people of one continent do not wish to make their secrets known to people of other continents. The excuse is "Westerners don't like the smell of coconut oil!"

Today we are going to focus on our hands. Beautiful, graceful and well-kept hands are an asset to everyone. Whether your nails are perfectly filed or are just polished half-heartedly can make all the difference about people's opinion about you.

How many times have you seen women with chipped nail polish and felt an instant feeling of half superior contempt? Let me admit it – being in high-powered jobs, where I needed to be perfectly groomed all the time, I learned very early that ladies looked straight at my nails and hands, when I found myself gesturing during meetings or presentations. And that is why the nail polish had to be perfect and hand maintenance had to be immaculate. White for choice, for professional working ladies, but if you are getting your hands ready for an informal tomorrow you can try all sorts of combinations and permutations to get beautiful color effects on your fingertips. Try something like a red base with a light blue or green second coat, covered with white to get a pretty and unusual affect. Do not be scared to experiment!

But who really has the time to remove one's old nail polish and freshen it up every night? The best time is of course at night just before going to sleep. Or when you are sitting in front of the television or when you are about to change your clothes, getting ready for bed after you have moisturized your face with the milk and salt!

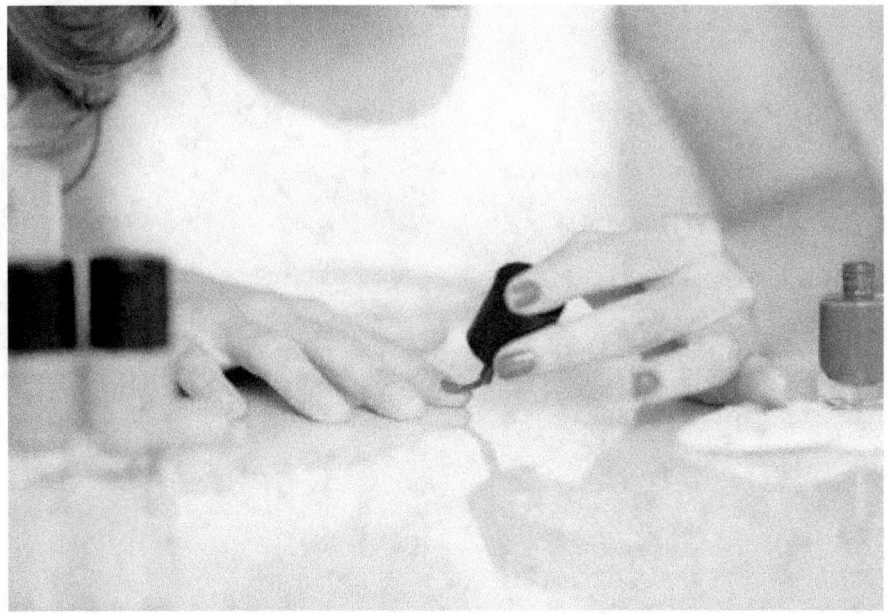

The easiest way to prevent your polish from chipping is to apply a nail base and then a layer of your favorite nail polish. The nail base is a transparent nail polish and when the first layer of nail polish dries, you go in for the second application.

Nail polish takes about 10 to 15 minutes to dry perfectly. If by any chance you do not have the time to spare, insert your fingertips in a bowl of ice cold water. Your nail polish will have set perfectly in about half a minute. Nevertheless, 15 minutes air drying solidifies it even better.

Moisturize your hands with almond oil, coconut oil, or wheat germ oil to keep them supple and well- toned.

Day 3

Today's the day of the coconut and the day when you are going to concentrate on hair care. This is the day when you are going to go hunting for fresh coconut juice. If you live in areas where you can get easy access to coconuts, you are lucky, because fresh coconut juice is supposed to be the best anti-dehydrating agent known to mankind. Doctors without access to medicines in typhoon hit coastal areas immediately put their patients on a coconut water diet so that they do not get infections through polluted water. Also, these people will not suffer from dehydration ever, even if they do not have access to oral rehydration solutions.

So now that you have got your coconut, you are going to apply that juice to your face, and also drink the coconut water. If you do not have access to coconut juice, you will need to make do with unrefined coconut oil. Apply it gently around your eyes and wherever you think that wrinkles are about to attack. Feel your skin soak up at the coconut oil, which is an excellent moisturizer and revitalizer.

Today is the day for hair care. Now let me admit it. One of the reasons why so many people in the Orient, have long hair is because they use mustard oil and coconut oil to condition their hair. Both of them have very powerful odors, but as I heard one rustic shepherd answer me, when I asked him how he managed to live up in the mountains for three months or more, without access to enough water for baths, he said, in the vernacular, something which is freely translated as – "everyone in our group smells the same, especially when we are around our sheep and goats. So I do not bother too much about how I smell!" Now that is a practical way of saying, it is no use being sensitive about powerful odors of oils when everybody around you has been slathering them all over their bodies, hair and faces.

If you can manage to get unrefined mustard oil – statuary warning – three times more strong odor than unrefined coconut oil – and have an hour free before you shampoo and shower, try rubbing it in your hair and scalp with your fingertips and over your body. This is very strong oil, so do not use it on your face for moisturizing. If you have a dandruff problem, add yogurt to the mustard oil, or to the coconut oil before you go in for this pre-shampoo conditioning. Keep this oil on for about 4 to 5 hours, so that it can soak into your roots completely. In Asia, normally this oil is applied on Saturday night, and left overnight.

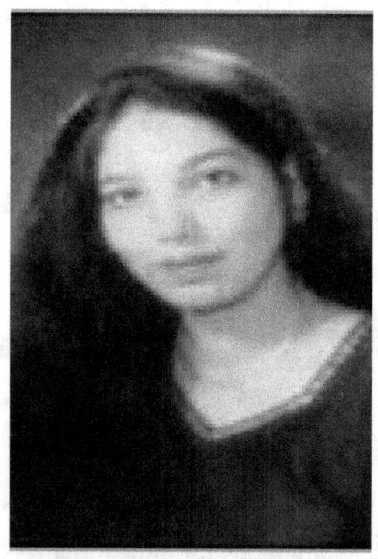

Let me admit it - My long shiny long hair is due to coconut oil massages as a child and mustard oil massages as an adult. Mustard oil prevents the greying of hair. (courtesy:DJS)

Now your immediate reaction is "come on, if I oil my hair at night and leave it so overnight, who is going to come here and wash the oily, greasy sheets, you? I don't think so."

Well, here is the solution. Dip a towel in hot water, wrap your hair into it and leave it alone for about 20 minutes. The moisture of the towel will immediately cause the oil to be absorbed directly into the scalp. No problem of greasy sheets. But, because I like my hair oiled for 7 to 8 hours overnight, I wrap it up in a towel turban on Saturday evening before shampooing on Sunday afternoon.

Some people recommend lemons as a good hair conditioner, but it has a tendency of bleaching the hair. So if you are a natural blonde, use lemons for hair conditioning. But if you are a brunette do not use this because this is going to lighten the color of your hair.

If you think that Henna is a wonderful hair conditioner, consider this fact. It may give a reddish color to your hair, but **you are not going to regain your natural hair color** when the Henna fades away. If you want to take the chance and experiment, do try this out. [Against my advice.] It is going to hasten the graying process of your hair.

Natural products are much better in the long run than artificial ones. We do have a wide range of shampoos, hair conditioners and other hair products promising all sorts of wonders, to keep your Crowning Glory silky and lustrous. But the chemicals used in their manufacture are going to have a detrimental effect on your hair. So try using natural shampoos like egg shampoos.

I use this egg shampoo whenever I want my hair to be squeaky clean and with that extra bounce.

Beat up an egg in ¼ cup coconut oil or olive oil. Massage this mixture through your hair and scalp and wash under a warm shower. Then wash your hair with two fistfuls of apple cider vinegar to get rid of the oily and sticky feel of oil. There you are- squeaky clean hair naturally.

In Victorian times, it was the practice of brushing one's hair 100 times every night before retiring. But then, they also had the practice of not having a regular head shampoo or even a bath. Washing your hair two times a week is going to eliminate the necessity of brushing it hundred times or more every night. There is a little loss of hair during the shampooing process and that is why no one can really afford to brush her hair 100 times every night in addition to shampooing. But if you really want to put a shine to it, take your favorite silk scarf and rub your hair with it gently. The static electricity so generated quite electrifies your hair and leaves it squeaky clean.

If you want to moisturize your hair even more, beat up an egg in some yogurt and apply it to your hair. Then wash your hair after 20 minutes.

Day 4: Today is papaya – on – the – skin and face masks day.

Eat as many organically grown fruit as you can, with papayas, playing a major role in your diet. I do hope you are still drinking either tomato or orange or cucumber juice as often as you can. A little slice of papaya or papaya pulp is needed to be applied all over your skin, but make sure that you do not rub hard. Some women say that orange juice can be used as a substitute, if they cannot find papaya. After all, it is also a juicy fruit and it is more readily available than papaya. Orange juice happens to be a suntrap while papaya's not. So if you want your skin beautifully sunburnt, do please apply orange juice. And then go out in the sun. And then come back home with a red peeling nose and a bad case of sunburn.

I use organic vinegar to alleviate the suffering caused due to sunburn. But just imagine that you have been neglecting your skin for a long time, and are suffering from a bad case of tanning and sunburn. You want to get back to the original stage of bleached skin without tan and sunburn. This process, which I am going to tell you, may seem to be a bit messy, but it is extremely effective. Not only does it to get rid of your sunburn and tan, but it keeps your skin soft too.

Before getting ready for your bath, add 2 tablespoons of your favorite moisturizing oil – wheat germ, almond or coconut oil – to four tablespoons full of oatmeal. If you have the time and the inclination, you can always add some rosewater [rosewater making process – please see appendix.] and glycerin to make up a smooth paste. Now apply this smooth paste on your face, hands and wherever you think of that there is sunburn.

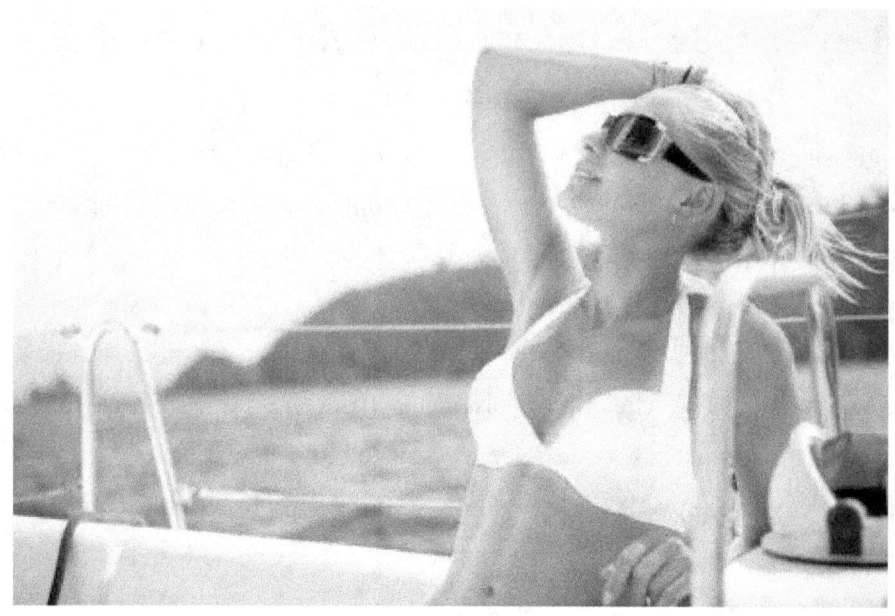

A suntan may look gorgeous on you now but it is ruining the texture of your skin.

Leave on for about three – five minutes and then gently wetting your hands begin to scrub off the paste. See the immediate of this mask. Some women insist on applying this mask made up of milk cream. But I have noticed that cream does not have the necessary consistency to rub off so smoothly. Besides, it takes anywhere from 10 to 20 minutes to dry and before you can rub it off.

Day 5

Today we are going to concentrate on skin problems. Today's the day of the poppy seed. The seeds of the Poppy have been used since ancient times to lend an almost fragile transparency to the skin. But the only problem is that they are so tiny that it is a bit of a problem to grind them to a paste. That is why slaves of aristocratic Roman, Egyptian and Greek ladies in olden times used to add milk to the Poppy seeds, before they ground them up in hand operated mortars.

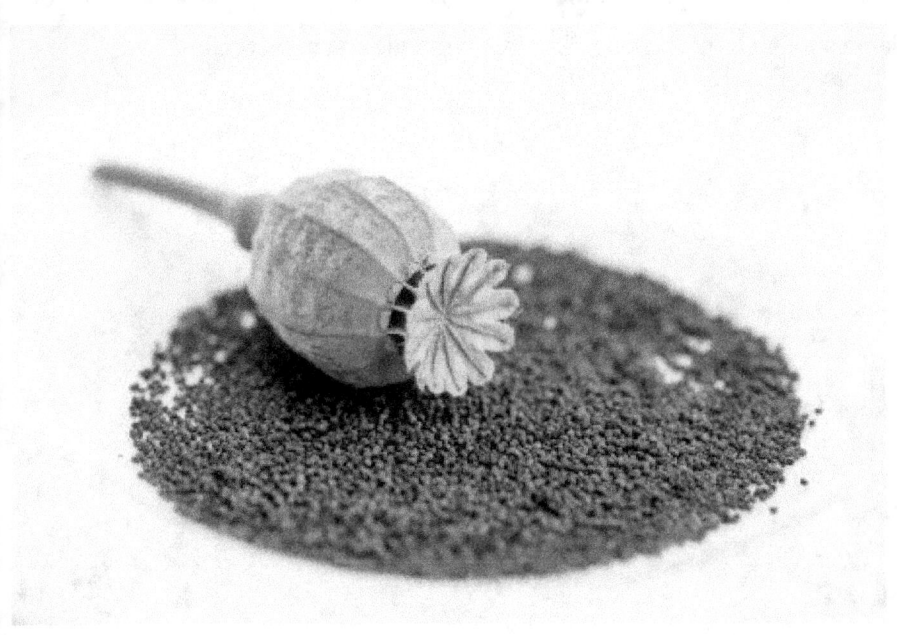

Grind the seeds with milk to a smooth paste. Luckily, we have grinders to grind them. Now apply it all over to your face and relax for 10 minutes. Wash with warm water. This is a once a week application, which is enough to leave your skin looking transparent and beautiful.

If you happen to be suffering from skin problems like pimples and blackheads, make a paste of brown mustard seeds with water and apply in the affected areas. These have been used since ancient times to dry up pimples and leave your skin scar free.

If that zit occurred right in time for your important day out, and it happens so often, all you have to do is grind some nutmeg with milk. Apply it on the trouble spot. This is going to have an immediate drying effect. We know that these spots have this remarkable tendency of coming out the night before you have to go out on an important social or special occasion when you want to look your best. Just dab a little of this paste upon the spot and saying "out out damn spot", go off to sleep. The spot will fade away overnight.

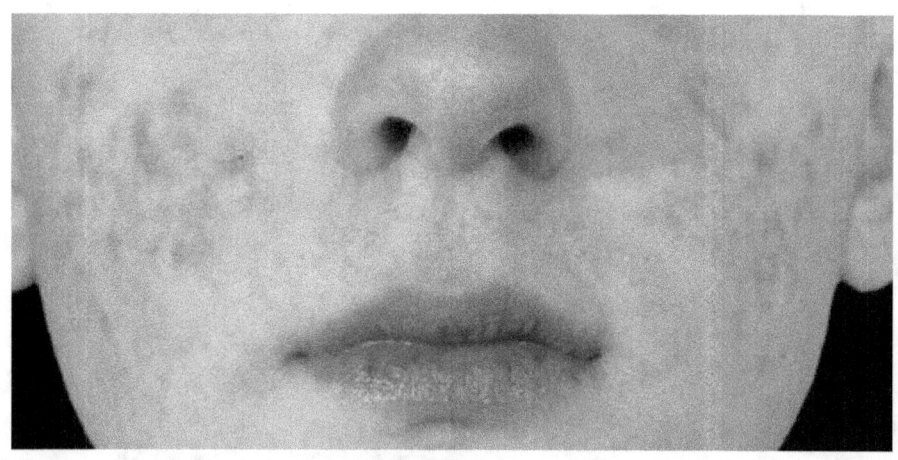

Is that you? Get rid of the scars with a turmeric/cream paste.

If you have a particularly spotty skin and you are worried about how best you can get rid of the scars, I would suggest a paste of freshly ground or original

turmeric powder and cream applied on this area. Leave it to dry and then slowly rub it off with warm water. The affected area skin is thus going to be exfoliated while the cream makes sure that it is still moisturized. Believe me, regular application of this paste every day will have new skin growing over the affected area. You may want to read more here-
http://voices.yahoo.com/turmeric-one-best-natural-beauty-products-1943958.html?cat=69

Day 6

Today's going to be the day of the Rose and the nose where we are going to pamper ourselves with fragrances and perfumes. One of the most popular and of course the most expensive of fragrances and perfumes is ittar- otherwise known as Otto-o'roses or Rose attar. Even though essential oils have been extracted through millenniums from flowers and spices, by condensation of flower petals or just boiling the flower petals in oil so that the oil gets infused with the essential oil, I am going to show you how to make an infusion and how to extract essential oils .

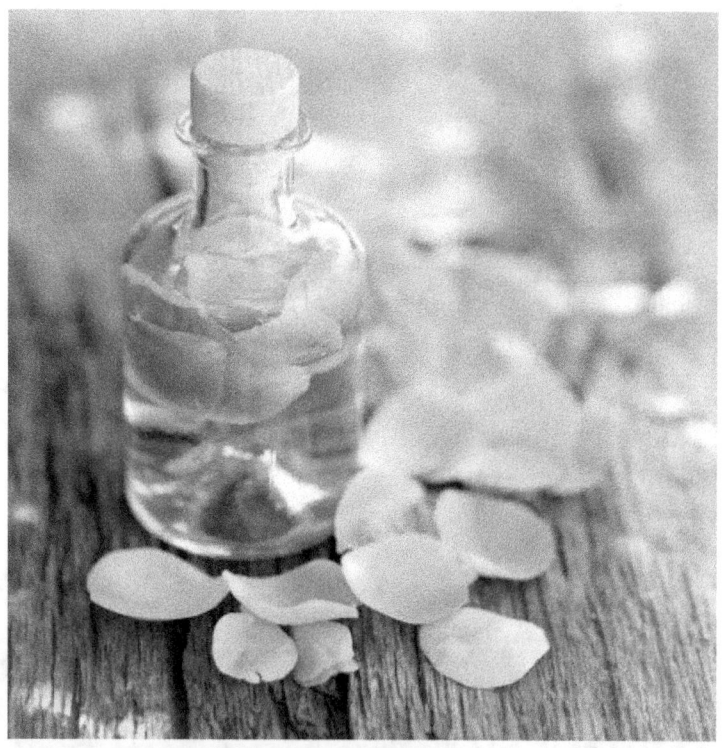

Rose essential oil. Use infusions as massage oil, bath oil, or just as a skin lotion.

Fill a large jar or a bottle with a good vegetable oil. Seriously speaking, almond oil, and wheat germ oil are good choices, but they are too expensive. So I use vegetable oil. Oil infusions are normally best made in the summertime, because one is fortunate enough to have an uninterrupted supply of sun.

Add red rose petals to the oil in just enough quantity to cover the bottom portion of a glass bottle. Two fistfuls of red rose petals are going to do very well, even though Marigold, geraniums lavender and Jasmine are good choices for infused oils. Do you know that that 10 g bottle of rose oil which you are buying for USD65 through companies which say that they are giving you pure rose oil extract has – in many cases – 90% of geranium oil and 10 percent of rose oil? So is not it worthwhile making your own rose oil, especially when you have access to lots of sun, rose flowers and a big glass jar?

The rose petals should not be packed tight. These petals will soon become brown in color. Remove them and add a fresh lot of petals. This process has to be repeated under the color of the oil shows a light red tint. It may take about 10 to 12 changes, but this is enough to capture the fragrance of the red rose. Decant the oil in a jar, and make sure that there is no vestige of petals remaining in the oil.

Now this oil can be used as a skin lotion or as a perfume in itself. Is not it much more soul satisfying to make your own natural perfume and skin lotion, rather than spending thousands of dollars on chemical-based brand name beauty products? Some other flowers like Marigold can be used as a good and effective lotion for tiny scratches, burns, cuts and wounds.

How to make an infusion?

All you have to do is to put some water on the boil and add two handfuls of petals in the water, let it bubble for about 15 minutes. I use Marigold flowers, and this gives the water a golden tint. I wash my face with this when I do not have cucumber juice cleansing lotion nearby. This is an extremely good, as stringent and gives your skin a golden glow.

It is now time to tackle the problem spots at the corner of your elbows, and the soles of your feet. The skin of your elbow corners can be made softer and smoother, just by massaging it with oil, after having taken a bath or shower.

A loofah or a good scrubber well soaped can be rubbed in clockwise direction to tackle the elbow corners. As for those painful cracks in your heels, you would need to rub them slowly with pumice stone.

Make sure your feet are quite well soaked and the skin tender before you rub off the dead cells. Do this gently; you do not want those cracks bleeding, do you? If they happen to be bleeding and painful, I would suggest making a poultice of crushed Neem leaves and apply it on the cracked heels, and then put on socks to keep them in place. Neem, which is indigenous in the Indian subcontinent is now growing in many parts of the world.

Learn more about the Neem here-
http://en.wikipedia.org/wiki/Azadirachta_indica

Day 7

Today's the day to rest and count your blessings. You are also going to do some physical exercises to look good but you need plenty of mental stimulus like being surrounded a beauty in the garden or among the flowers, just to take deep breaths which are full of peace and which will help set your mind, your body and spirit at ease.

Try walking in the lap of nature when you are feeling particularly sad. The best revitalizing exercise is of course lying down on the green grass, just braving the insects and midges for about 5 to 10 minutes setting your eyes and taking deep breaths. Let nature help you regain peace by soothing you. Nature is the world's greatest healer and you will feel your tiredness just fade away into nothing.

A woman normally feels incapable of thinking herself good-looking if she is not mentally, emotionally and spiritually happy. You owe it to yourself to spend at least five minutes of your busy 24 hours schedule to say to yourself – "think beautiful, I am beautiful. I like myself. I like everything about me. Today's a beautiful day. I have faith in tomorrow. Tomorrow is also going to be a good day for me and my family and the people around me." These are positive thoughts, and believe me, when you are thinking them when you are lying down on the lawn you are going to find these thoughts resonating throughout your body and spirit.

Some of the most beautiful women can make themselves look ordinary, and vice versa by thinking so. This is a proven fact.

These positive strokes are necessary to keep your self-respect, self-esteem, pride and a healthy state of mind right and intact. And do not let anybody else persuade you otherwise.

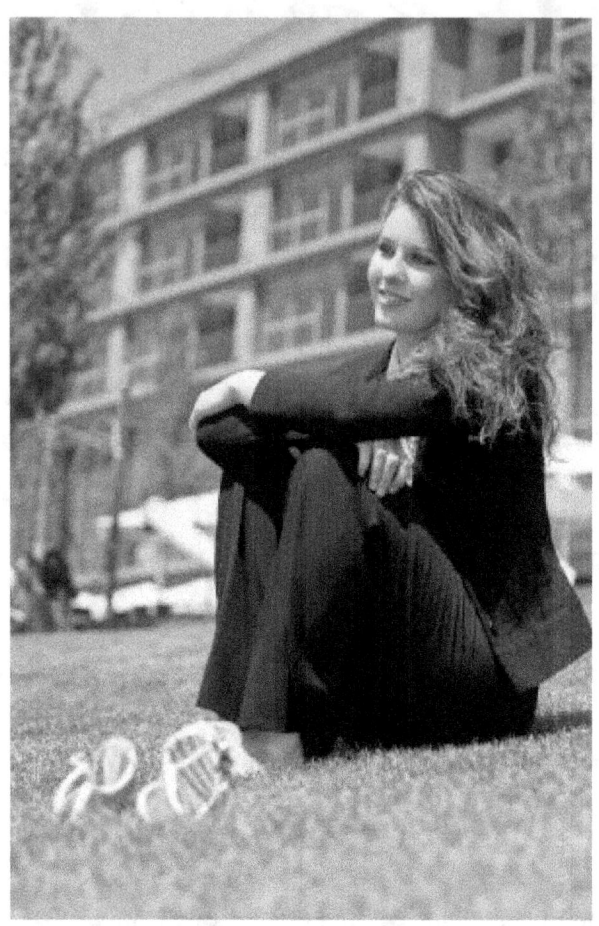

A person does not love himself or herself and has some sort of inverted guilt complex, if he thinks that cherishing and cossetting oneself is something which he should deny himself. This definitely does not come under the seven deadly sins. It is not a sin to make yourself look good and feel good about yourself.

I remember an instance when I was talking about the same cherishing oneself idea to a group of ladies, who looked at me askance, and some had expressions of horror and dismay. According to them, this beautification of oneself for a wife and mother, and especially one in the older age group would have people around them ridiculing them. I was shocked when I heard this. But remember, be thou as pure as the driven snow, thou shalt not escape calumny. There is going to be some person, somewhere, who is too lazy to take care of herself or himself. And she/he definitely does not like you looking good because he/she thinks you are trying to gain attention with all that pampering yourself. You cannot do anything about their mental state and their thought processes. So do not get stressed out when you are confronted with such narrow minded lumps of humanity.

Women also use this stupid idea as an excuse that XYZ shall not like it if I pamper myself a bit. Well, they can now go and tell XYZ that they are not spending money on chemical cosmetics, but are growing beautiful naturally.

Besides this, XYZ shall see a remarkable and visible difference when you quietly try this six-day beauty treatment starting right now.

Appendix

How to Make Rosewater

How to make Rose water

Rosewater is normally available in markets at exorbitant prices, but in India, anybody with access to the red rose – Rosa Damascena and a little bit of time enjoys making Rosewater at home. This Rosewater is used in cosmetics, as well as in cookery to impart the flavor of the Rose to your meal or to your skin.

Ingredients needed- 1 Cup Rose petals – 12 to 14 flowers.

2 cups water

Lots of ice.

A huge cooking pan – pan number one – with lid in which another pan – pan number two – can be placed comfortably.

Rosewater is just a matter of distillation. Put a wire stand in pan number one, on which you are going to stand the other pan number two. The condensed Rosewater is going to fall into pan number two.

Place the petals at the bottom of the pan number one. Now, cover the petals with water. Place pan number two on the wire stand. Now take the lid and place it upside down on pan number one, thus effectively covering the Rose petals, pan number two and the water. The Rose water is going to condense when you place the blocks and chunks of ice on the inverted lid.

You are going to have a cupful of precious distilled Rosewater, after 25 minutes of slow steaming of the Rose petals.

Precautions – remember to have enough of water to cover the Rose petals. Also, it should not be of such a large quantity, that it displaces the wire stand.

This cooled water is now pure Rosewater. Pour it in a sterilized glass bottle. Use it to your heart's content. You may see a little bit of oil swimming over the surface of the water. This is Rose oil, and is even more precious. So if you used lots of petals in a larger pan, you may find even more Rose oil.

Author Bio

Dueep Jyot Singh is a Management and IT Professional who managed to gather Postgraduate qualifications in Management and English and Degrees in Science, French and Education while pursuing different enjoyable career options like being an hospital administrator, IT,SEO and HRD Database Manager/ trainer, movie scriptwriter, theatre artiste and public speaker, lecturer in French, Marketing and Advertising, ex-Editor of Hearts On Fire (now known as Solctice) Books Missouri USA, advice columnist and cartoonist, publisher and Aviation School trainer, ex- moderator on Medico.in, banker, student councilor ,travelogue writer … among other things! One fine morning, she decided that she had enough of killing herself by Degrees and went back to her first love -- writing. It's more enjoyable! She already has 38 published academic and 14 fiction- in- different- genre books under her belt.

When she is not designing websites or making Graphic design illustrations for clients who want Walt Disney, Norman Rockwell , JJ Grandville or Hed Kandy type illustrations, she is busy browsing in old bookshops for antique books,-she has a mouthwatering collection of priceless First editions and rare books…including R.L. Stevenson, O.Henry, Dornford Yates, Maurice Walsh, C.N.Williamson, and the crown of her collection- Dickens "The Old Curiosity Shop," and so on… Just call her "Renaissance Woman") - collecting herbal remedies, making one of a kind creations in Irish Crochet and Aran knitting, acting like Universal Helping Hand/Agony Aunt, or escaping to her dear mountains for a bit of exploring, collecting herbs and plants , trekking, and rappelling.

Check out some of the other JD-Biz Publishing books

Gardening Series on Amazon

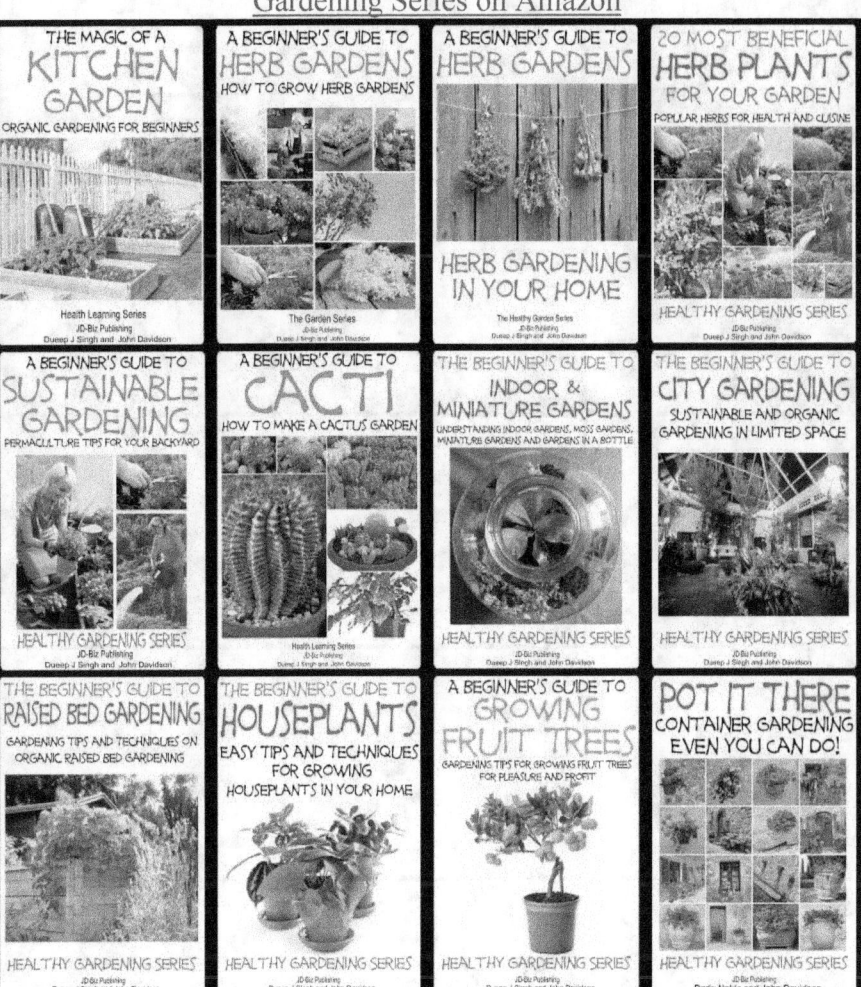

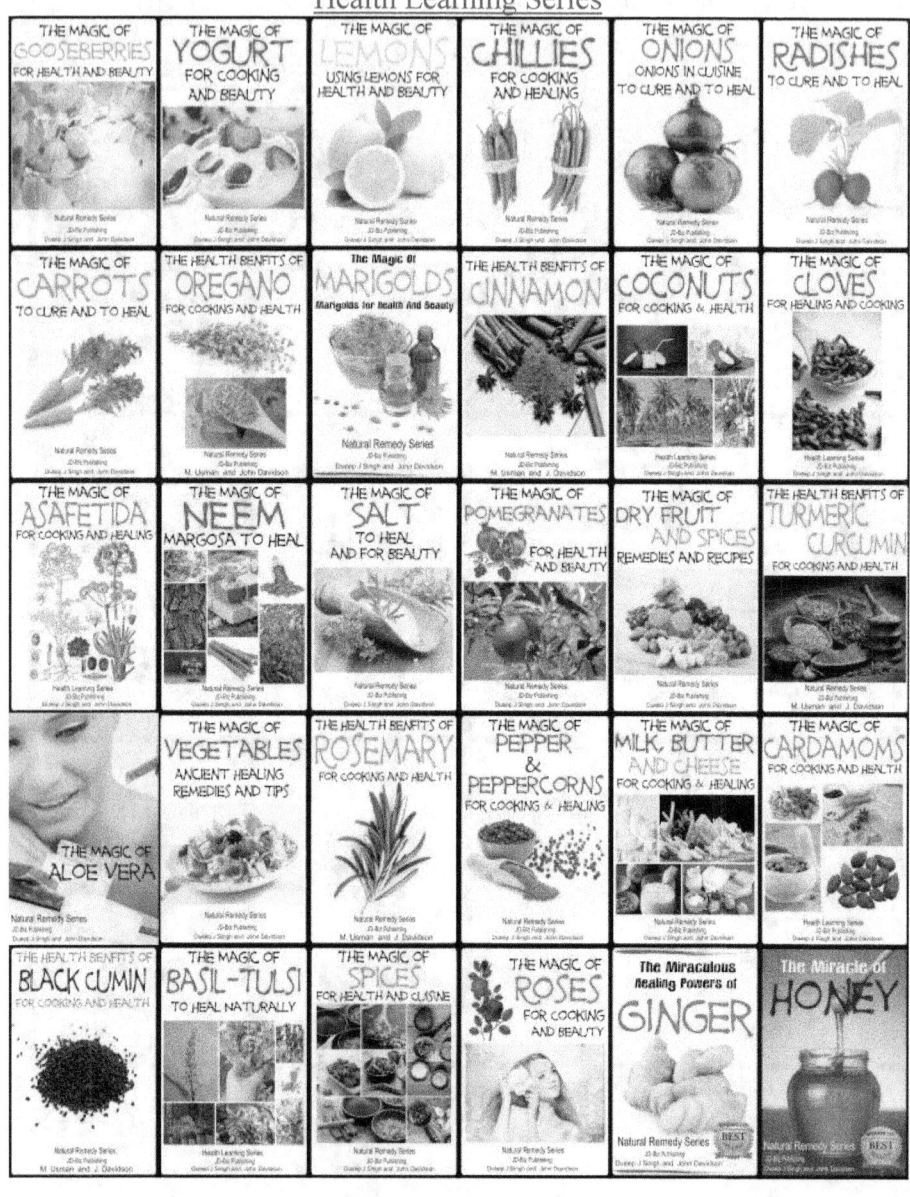

Country Life Books

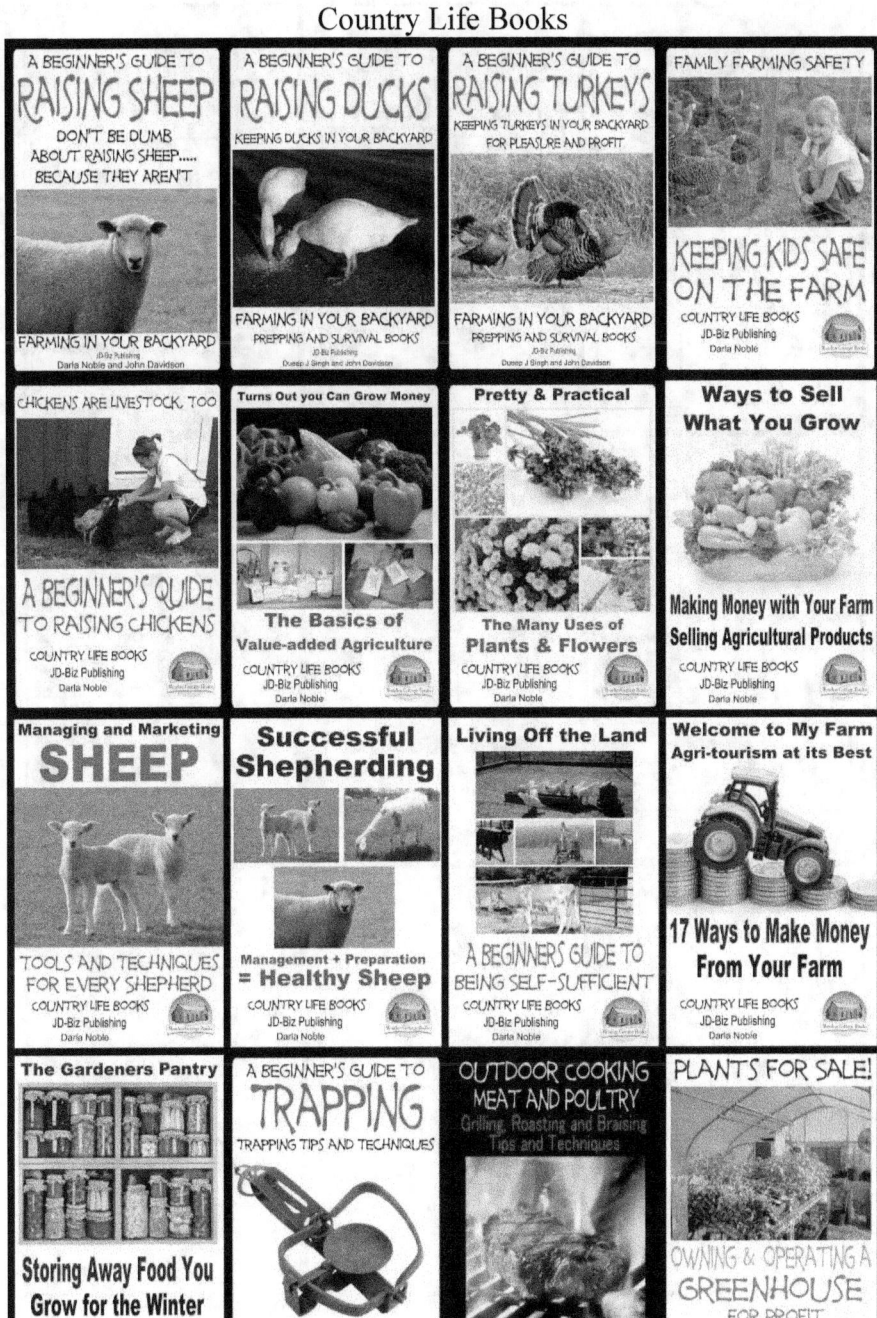

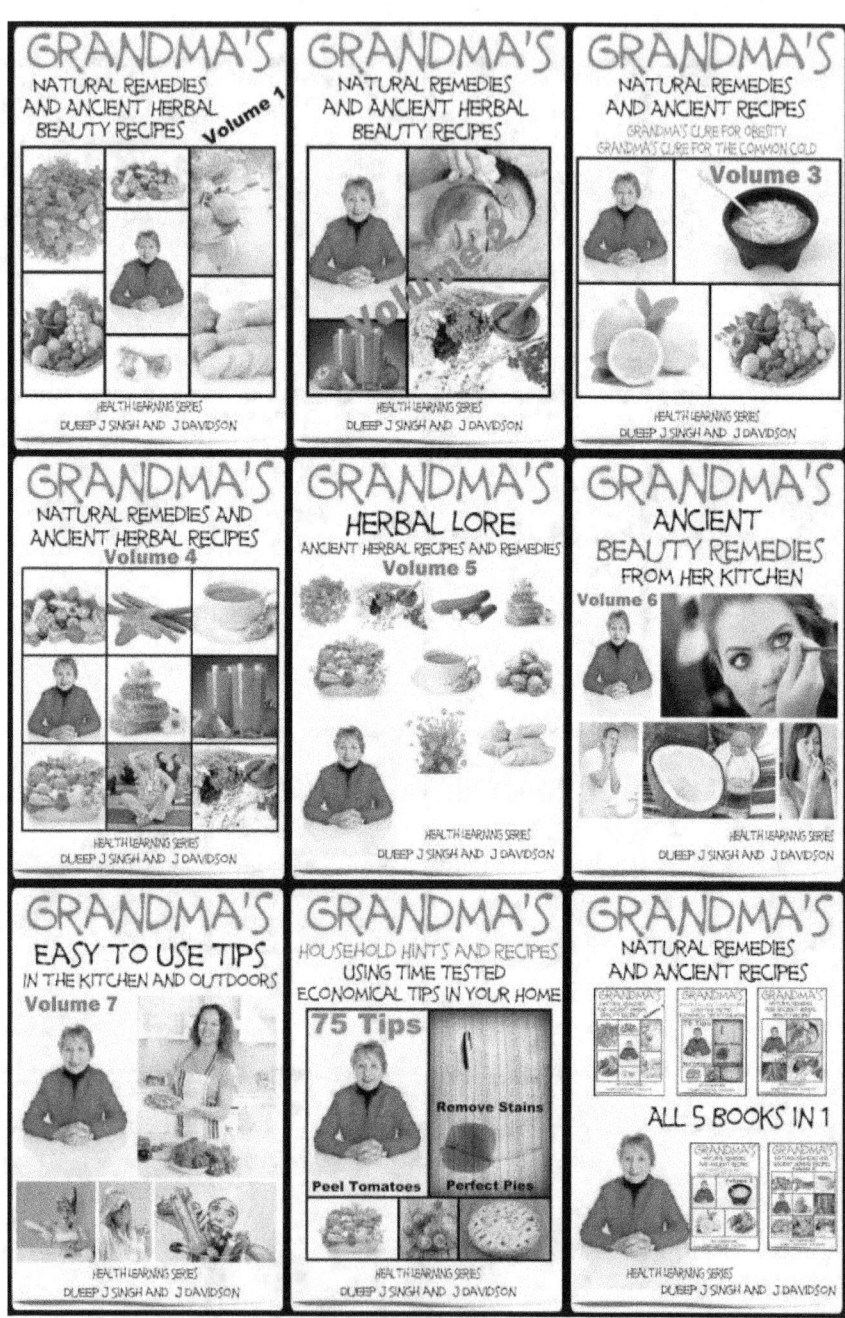

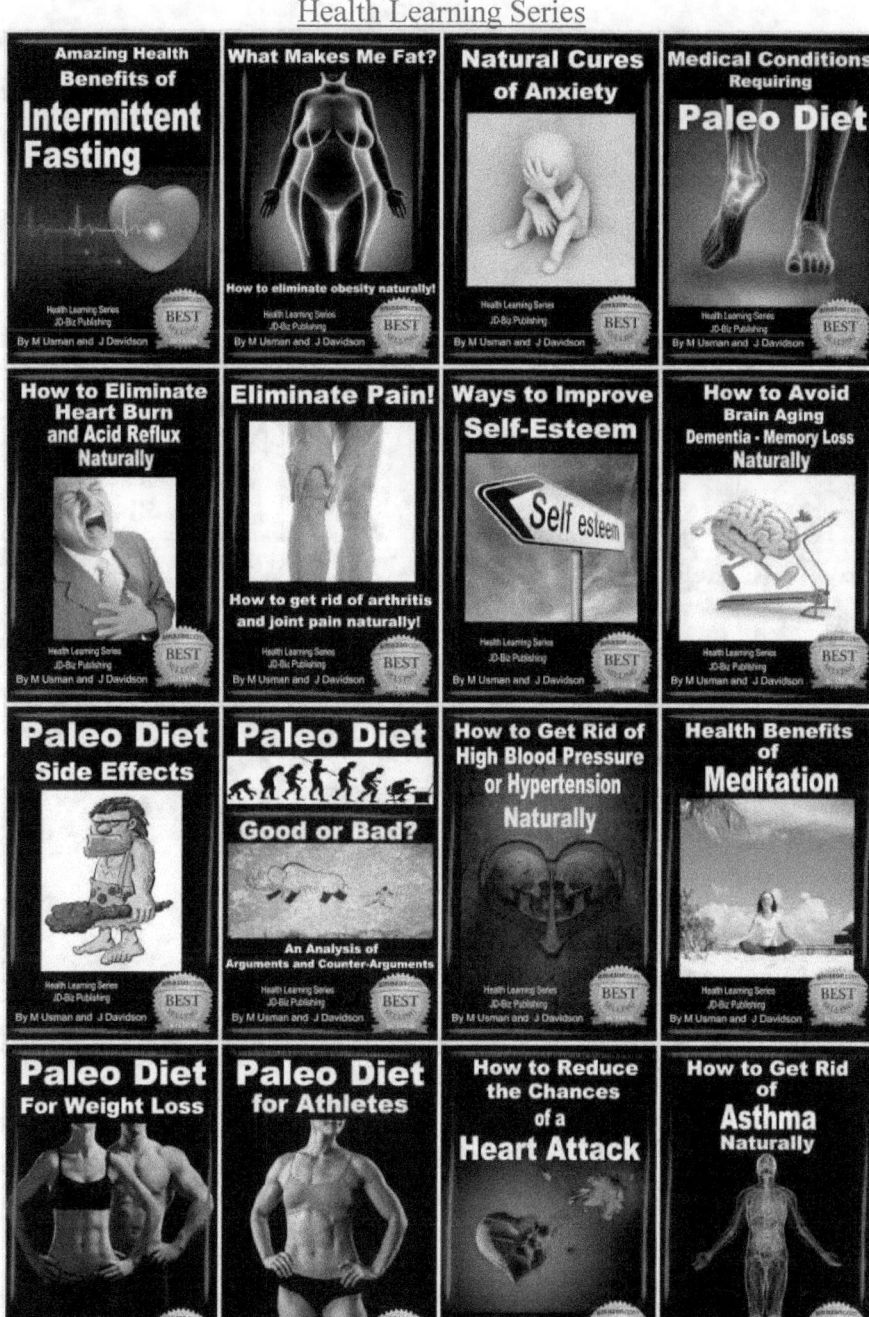

Amazing Animal Book Series

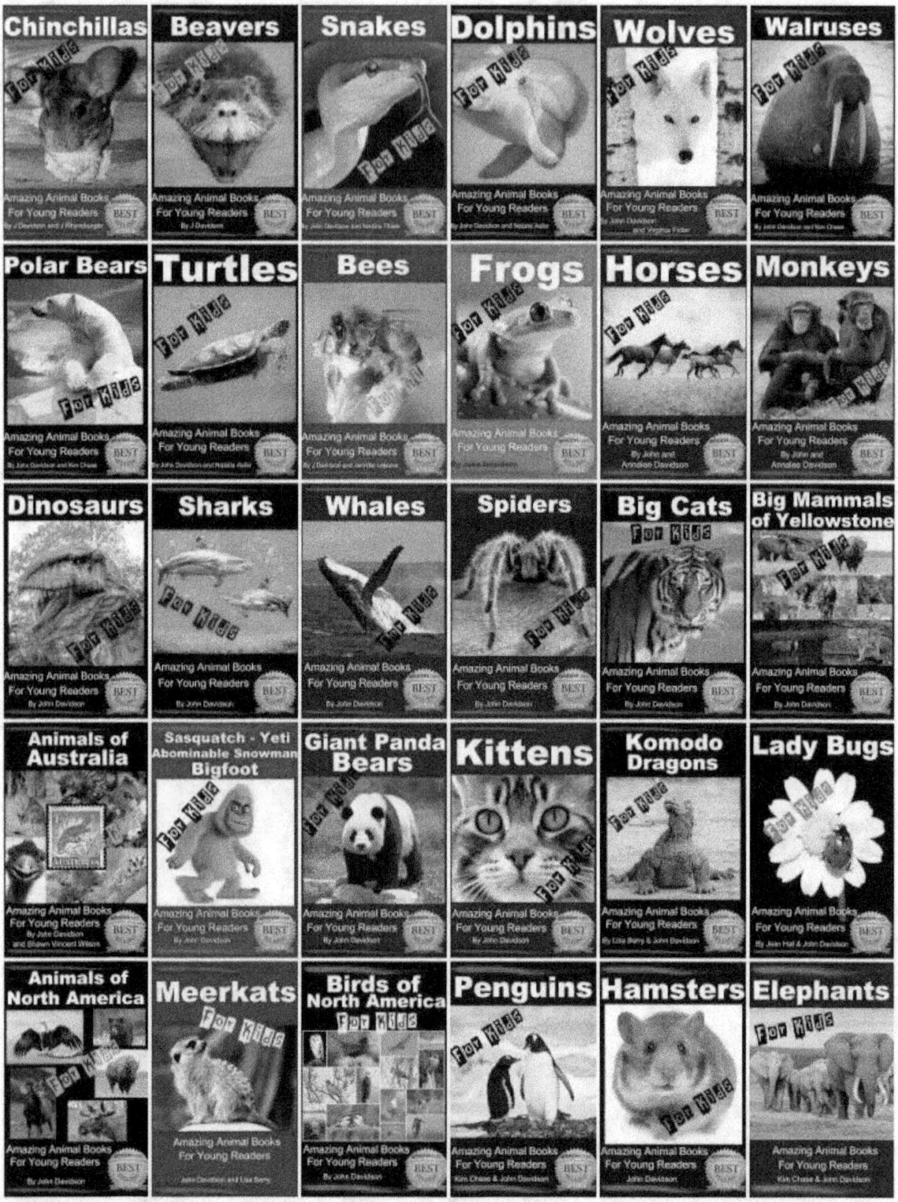

Learn To Draw Series

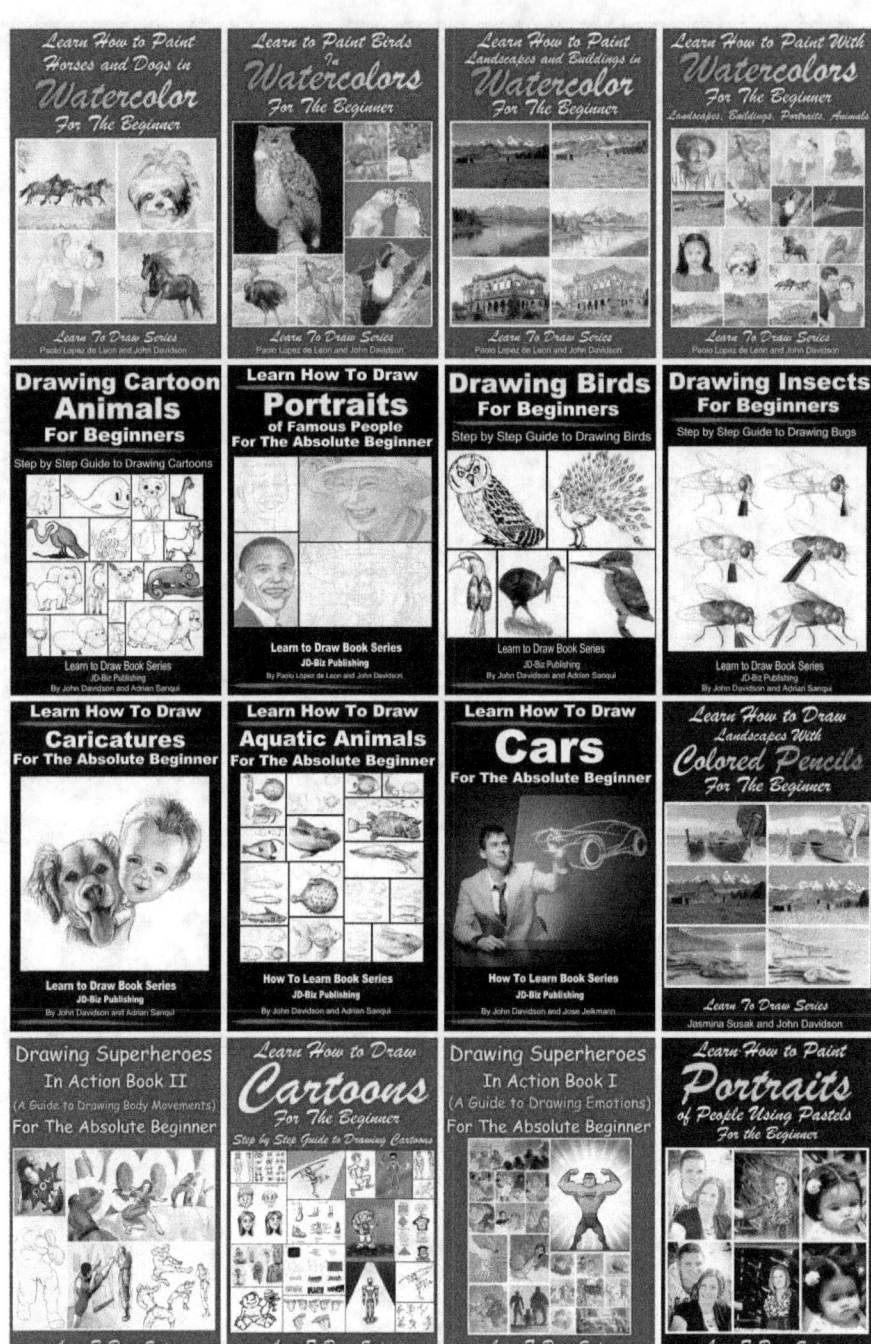

How to Build and Plan Books

Entrepreneur Book Series

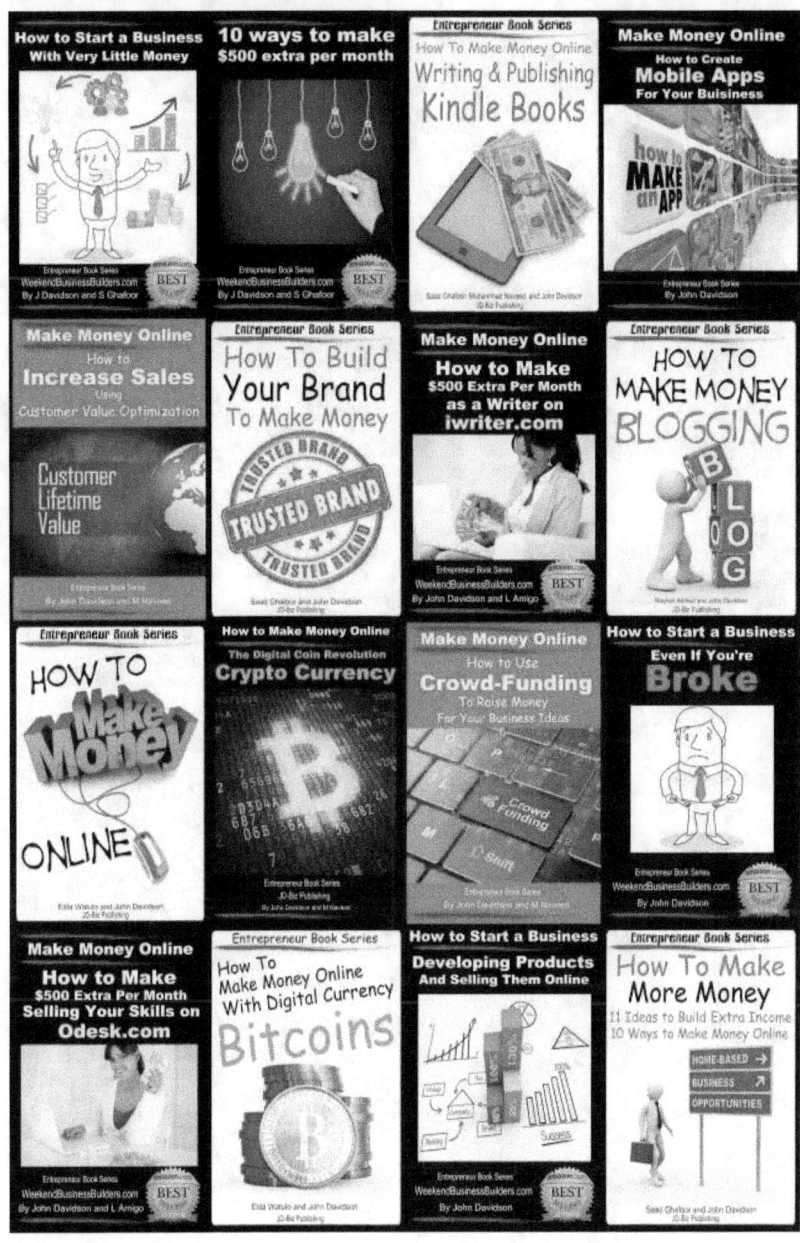

Our books are available at

1. Amazon.com

2. Barnes and Noble

3. Itunes

4. Kobo

5. Smashwords

6. Google Play Books

Download Free Books!

http://MendonCottageBooks.com

Publisher

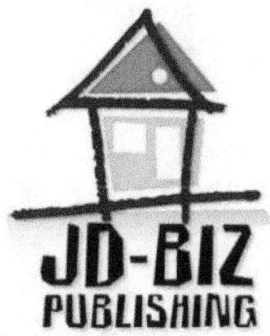

JD-Biz Corp

P O Box 374

Mendon, Utah 84325

http://www.jd-biz.com/

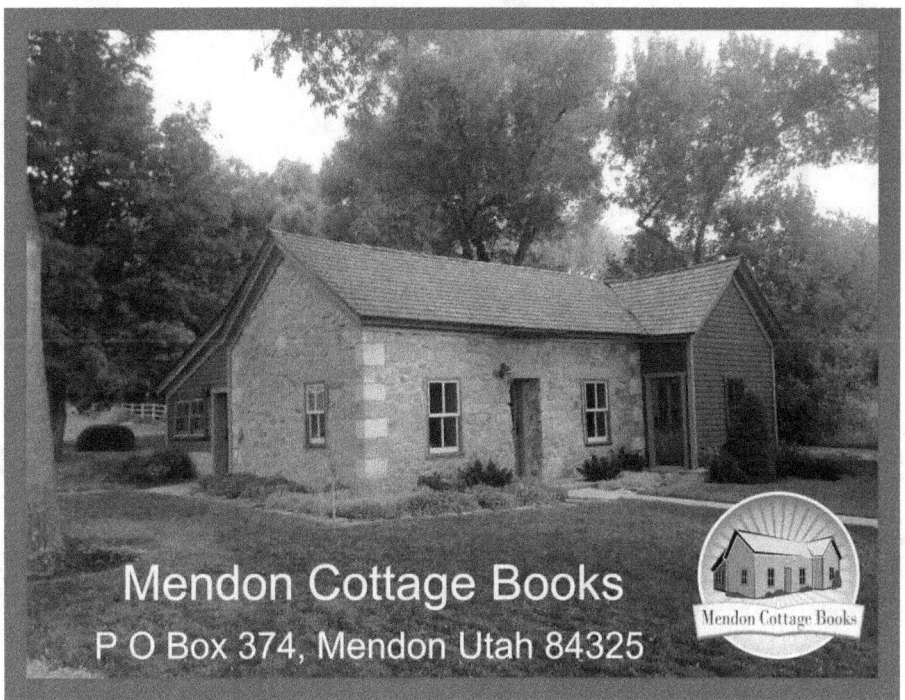

Mendon Cottage Books

P O Box 374, Mendon Utah 84325